120 Organic Skin Care Recipes

Homemade Aromatherapy Essential Oil Recipes for Complete Natural Body Care

Make Your Own Body Scrubs, Body Butters, Shampoos,

Lotions, Bath Recipes and Masks

(Organic body ... homemade body butter, body care recipes)

JACQUELINE S MENDEZ

Limit of Liability

The information in this book is solely for informational
purposes, not as a medical instruction to replace the advice of
your physician or as a replacement for any treatment prescribed
by your physician. The author and publisher do not take
responsibility for any possible consequences from any treatment,
procedure, exercise, dietary modification, action or application of
medication which results from reading or following the
information contained in this book.

If you are ill or suspect that you have a medical problem, we
strongly encourage you to consult your medical, health, or other
competent professional before adopting any of the suggestions
in this book or drawing inferences from it.

This book and the author's opinions are solely for informational
and educational purposes. The author specifically disclaims all
responsibility for any liability, loss, or risk, personal or otherwise
which is incurred as a consequence, directly or indirectly, of the
use and application of any of the contents of this book.

ISBN-13: 978-1544761541

ISBN-10: 1544761546

DEDICATION

To all who desire to live life to the fullest!

TABLE OF CONTENT

INTRODUCTION

In the world today, the regular person lathers, slathers sprays and rubs an average of ten kinds of skin care products on the body on a daily basis. Unfortunately the skin is exposed to approximately one hundred and thirty different chemicals regularly absorbed by the skin.

Beauty, cosmetics and skin care companies with the Food and Drug Administration makes us believe that these chemicals are not harmful; on the contrary, if we keep exposing our skins to many of these chemicals over time, they are harmful to health.

The buildup of these many chemicals on a daily basis from the spray of deodorants, perfumes and so on, a small dab here and there, to make up on the regular woman should be considered. The dangers posed by these chemicals over a period cannot be fully ascertained by anyone.

Some chemicals are known to have great side effects and dangers. These chemicals are found in several artificial fragrances, for instance, Phthalates is a chemical known to be a hormone disruptor that causes sperm damage, birth defects, infertility, and male babies feminization.

The Environmental Working Group records nearly ninety percent of over ten thousand beauty, cosmetics and skin care ingredients that are known to the FDA and have not been tested to be unharmful by the Food and Drug Administration, Cosmetic Ingredient Review, or any other Institution that is publicly accountable.

Candidly, manufacturers are careful not to harm their customers, at least nobody drops dead after the use of a body wash or mascara wand. But on the long run, we should be careful with the use of complex chemicals with no known dangers or hazards and that haven't been evaluated to be safe. The European Union banned over one thousand beauty, cosmetics, personal and skin care ingredients on the basis that they may be causes of reproductive ills, birth defects or cancers. In the U.S only ten of these ingredients have been banned.

To be on the safe side, it becomes imperative that we green our beauty routine by

1. Simplifying our choices of beauty products. Most beauty companies cannot deliver on the promises they make, so do not be deceived by cosmetic adverts. Many of these high brow fancy beauty products would never deliver on turning the tide of growing older. My recommendations for eye creams, for instance, is to keep everything simple since eye creams hardly have varying formulations from the regular face moisturizer; the necessary things needed is a toner, basic cleanser, broad spectrum sunscreen and moisturizer to keep in beautiful shape. Everything other thing is just a cover.

2. Go for zero-fragrance products. Fragrance mixtures usually contain several toxic chemicals used in production, and these companies are not required by federal laws to

state any of the chemicals used in the ingredients. These pose hidden threats and dangers to health. Stay away from labels that have "parfum" or "fragrance" written on them.

3. Be certain that Natural isn't stylishly synthetic. Carefully watch and examine any beauty product you may consider.

Many beauty products are filled with toxic chemicals. And the fact that natural and all natural are written on the label doesn't necessarily mean it is the truth; as these words are not terms that are regulated in any way.

4. What are the company values of the skin care product you are considering? Visit the website of the company, look out for the values and philosophy of the company; this can be a life-saver. Check out if it has a signed compact for cosmetics that are safe and a promise to take out any chemical considered harmful and a threat to life from the list of ingredients and find unharmful replacements, does it test on animals, for instance? All these should be considered before making a buy.

5. Go for a recyclable packaging that you are sure is non-toxic. Glass is a great option as it is recyclable and wouldn't leach toxins into the skin care product contained inside. Some plastics are harmful and poisonous to the body when used as packaging for skin care products. Few of these plastics are safe and recyclable. For instance, (HDPE) high density

polyethene known by the recycling code #2, and (PET) Polyethylene terephthalate, #1, are believed to be safe and very often accepted by the municipal curbside recycling programs. Avoid plastics that cause health and environmental hazards from manufacture, use and to disposal.

6. Avoid Petrochemicals. Beauty or Skin care products that have petrolatum, paraffin and mineral oil written on the label are a no go area! Because many byproducts of petroleum often times have varying degrees of cancer-containing impurities.

7. Go for beauty and skin care products that are organic. An ingredient grown without pesticides or fertilizers is known as Organic. They are healthier for both our bodies and the earth. Biodynamic methods of farming are used to grow organic ingredients. To be certain that the beauty, skin and body care product you are considering to buy is biodynamic, check for the stamp of approval of Demeter U.S.A on the label.

8. Be the manufacturing company. The best safety precaution to be taken is to make your own beauty, skin and body care products.

It saves you a lot, financially, packaging, and you can be certain it is preservatives and toxic-chemical free.

9. Avoid trends that are exotic. They are not always as they seem, and most times they end up becoming harmful to us or the environment.

10. Be beautiful all round by staying healthy. You don't need the extreme to look beautiful, resorting to surgeries, combinations of lotions and potions to become beautiful. Exercising and Dieting are also a key factor when following a skin care routine. Watch what you eat, eat right

and work out properly, and you can be certain that toxins will be flushed out instead of it messing up your beautiful skin.

FIGURES YOU SHOULD KNOW

1. The average woman will ingest 4 lbs. of lipstick over a lifetime.

2. Only 1155 ingredients out of 10,500 used in beauty, skin and body care products have been publicly evaluated and recorded by the U.S government to be unharmful to the population.

3. The U.S government banned only 10 ingredients that used in cosmetics.

4. The European Union has banned over 1,110 of these ingredients and chemicals.

5. The amount of beauty, skin, personal and body care products said to have at least one cancer causing chemical is placed at 20%

6. Only 600 of the several beauty and cosmetics company have signed the compact for safe cosmetics.

7. Cosmetics and beauty products that contains the possible cancer causing impurity 1,4-dioxane are placed at 22%.

8. On a yearly basis, the amount spent on cosmetic surgeries, hair care, skin care, diet products, health clubs and fragrances is placed at $160 billion US dollars.

CHAPTER ONE - ORGANIC SKIN AND BEAUTY RECIPES FOR THE FACE (EYE SERUMS, FACE BRIGHTENER, TONER, FOUNDATION, FACE WASH, CLEANSERS....)

Homemade witch hazel makeup remover recipe

Sleeping in makeup is a nightmare; eventually you get up in the morning feeling so out of sorts and itchy. This recipe is easy and quick to help remove make up naturally with your own homemade make up remover pads.

You just wipe off the makeup and you can go to bed happy

Ingredients

4 oz. glass container with cover

1-2 tbsps witch hazel

1/2 tbsp liquid castile soap

1-2 vitamin E capsules

2 drops tea tree oil

30 cotton pads

2 tbsps water

Instructions

1. In a small bowl, combine the witch hazel, liquid castile soap, vitamin E capsules, and tea tree oil together.

NOTE: Using a sterile-pin, pierce the Vit. E capsules to get out the oil.

2. Place 25 cotton pads into the glass container and toss the bowl's mixture over the pads.

3. Lock the lid in place and shake vigorously.

NOTE: If any of the liquid mixture remains, add more pads until all the liquid mixture becomes absorbed.

4. Turn the pads over and add the 2 tbsps of water and lock the lid back in place.

5. Keep in a cool, dry place.

6. Apply by wiping your face with the makeup remover pads. Avoid the eyes area when wiping.

NOTE: This natural make up remover doesn't need to be washed off or rinsed after use.

TIP: You can put a little amount of warmed coconut oil in your hand and rub gently on your eye region, including your eye lashes using regular cotton pads to wipe away. You don't need to wash off or rinse.

NOTE: You can tweak it a little for your skin type. The Vitamin E oil works perfectly for a skin that is oily, and the tea tree oil will fix incessant skin breakouts. A 4 oz jelly jar would do well for packaging, just find anything that is not too tall and has enough room for your cotton pads.

Homemade turmeric skin brightener

This recipe is an easy homemade skin brightener that doesn't cost so much to make. It will rid your skin of age and sun spots. It also help to prevent diseases like cancer of the skin and it has anti inflammatory properties. It is known to reduce face pigmentation, pimples and acne.

Ingredients

1 tablespoon of hard coconut oil

1 tablespoon organic lemon juice

1/4 teaspoon organic turmeric

1 tablespoon of raw and organic honey

Organic witch hazel

Instructions

1. Combine hard coconut oil, lemon juice, turmeric and raw organic honey together, in a small container.

2. Mix thoroughly to combine.

3. Apply to the face, and leave for 10-15 minutes.

NOTE: Apply cream once in a week.

4. Wash off and rinse your face with warm water.

5. Spray witch hazel on your face, and then moisturize your skin as you would with your normal beauty routine.

Super All-Natural Anti Wrinkle Cream

Serves as an anti wrinkle, anti aging cream, also works wonders to remove scars.

Ingredients

3 teaspoons rosehip seed oil

2 teaspoons jojoba oil

3 teaspoons tamanu oil

3/4 teaspoon vegetable based emulsifying wax

3/4 teaspoon beeswax

1/2 teaspoon evening primrose oil

5 teaspoons matcha green tea

1 1/2 teaspoon aloe vera

1 1/2 teaspoon witch hazel

3-5 drops of peppermint essential oil

5-8 drops lavender essential oil

1/2 teaspoon wheatgerm oil

Instructions

1. Combine emulsifying wax, jojoba oil and beeswax together into a bowl.

2. Transfer into a double boiler and melt over medium low heat.

3. Once fully melted, take off from heat.

4. Transfer mixture into a refrigerator to semi-solidify.

5. Whisk wheat germ oil, primrose oil, tamanu oil and rosehip seed oil together in another bowl.

6. Transfer into an electric blender to blend.

7. Meanwhile, combine green tea, aloe vera, witch hazel, peppermint essential and lavender essential oil together in another bowl. Stir to combine well.

8. Pour green tea mixture in to the blender in a slow and steady stream at the highest speed of the blender.

9. Blend until blender mixture emulsifies completely.

10. Store in a jar.

DIY Moisturizing Eye Serum

Ingredients

2 tsps jojoba oil

2 tsps avocado oil

2 tsps apricot kernel oil

Instructions

1. Combine ingredients into a dropper bottle.

2. Cover bottle shake well to mix.

3. To apply, drop a tiny drop on your palms and use ring finger to apply to the skin area around the eye.

NOTE: Avoid putting serum to the eyes, eye lids or lashes directly or very near the eyes. It could irritate the eye.

4. Apply once a day at night.

5. Refrigerate.

Daily French Green Clay Bar

Ingredients

1/3 cup French green clay

1 tablespoon zinc oxide

1/3 cup kaolin clay

2 tablespoons witch hazel

1/8 teaspoon allantoin, if desired

8 grams melted shea butter

2 tablespoons aloe vera juice

Silicone mold

Instructions

1. Combine the dry ingredients together in a mixing bowl.

2. Whisk ingredients in the mixing bowl; slowly mix in the liquid ingredients.

3. After mixing well, knead until a sticky and stiff paste consistency is reached.

4. Transfer paste into the mold and smoothen the top. Set aside to 2-3 days to dry completely.

5. Turn mold over and place on a wire rack to dry completely for about a week.

6. Wash your face and wet the soap slightly.

7. Apply the wet side of the soap on your face.

NOTE: If the bar dries out, just wet again.

8. Leave it on your face to dry out for few minutes before you rinse off with a moist towel.

9. Apply argan oil after rinse off.

Homemade Natural Foundation with Sunscreen

Ingredients

Jojoba carrier oil

Cocoa butter

Shea butter

Vitamin E

Beeswax

Ground cinnamon

Zinc oxide (uncoated, non-nano, non-micronized)

Cocoa powder

Instructions:

1. Combine shea butter, jojoba, cocoa butter, vitamin E and beeswax in a bowl.

2. Stir to combine well.

3. Transfer and melt in a double boiler over medium low heat. Stirring frequently.

4. Take off from heat once mixture has melted completely.

5. Set aside for 5 minutes.

6. Measure in zinc oxide, and cinnamon, mixing to incorporate.

7. Measure in little cocoa powder and stir.

NOTE: Stir in little cocoa powder amounts in successions, stirring each time and comparing with your wrist color.

Stop adding extra cocoa powder when the mixture reaches your desired color consistency.

8. Transfer into a container and set aside to cool.

9. Coat lightly when applying.

Silk Face Mask with Luxurious Green Tea

This face mask refreshes and cleanses and helps to smoothen your face. Leaving your face firm with rich ingredients used in the recipe.

Ingredients

1 tablespoon aloe juice

1/4 teaspoon silk peptides, powder, or amino acids

1 teaspoon green tea extract or matcha powder

5 drops jojoba oil

4–6 teaspoon French green clay

Instructions

1. In a small dish, toss in the aloe juice.

2. Whisk in the silk and green tea into the aloe juice in the dish.

3. Measure in the clay slowly, 1 tsp per time, and whisk until a creamy and thick consistency is reached.

4. Measure in jojoba oil and whisk.

5. To apply, rub a rich amount of the mask on your face.

6. Leave for 20 minutes until mask begins to dry.

7. Wash off and apply argan oil to your face.

Homemade Clarifying and Toning Foaming Facewash

This recipe helps to tone and clarify the skin. It contains all-natural ingredients that are very gentle and would help to maintain the natural balance of your skin.

Ingredients

1 cup previously boiled or filtered water, (at room temperature)

5 tsps jojoba oil or another facial oil of choice

1/4 cup liquid castile soap

1 tsp tea tree oil

2 tbsps raw honey

10 drops rosemary essential oil

15 drops lavender essential oil

Instructions

1. In a small bowl, measure in water, soap, jojoba oil, raw honey, tea tree oil, lavender essential oil and rosemary essential oil.

NOTE: Add the ingredients in the written order in step 1, don't mix up the arrangements

2. Carefully stir mixture until well combined.

NOTE: The honey and castile soap will make the mixture look cloudy.

3. Transfer mixture into a foaming soap dispenser.

4. Apply facial wash once daily before bed time.

NOTE: Castile soap can be really concentrated. Do not use more than 1-2 pumps at a go. Do not use recipe for more than one month.

5. Shake well before each use.

NOTE: You can slightly adjust ingredients to suit your skin type. For a drier skin use lesser castile soap and more oil or water.

Witch Hazel Facial Toner Recipe with Vitamin C

Ingredients

1/2 teaspoon natural Vitamin C Powder

8 drops lavender essential oil, if desired.

1/4 cup witch hazel extract

Instructions

1. Mix vitamin C powder, witch hazel extract and the essential oil.

2. Mix well until well combined.

3. Transfer ingredients into a dropper bottle, glass bottle or spray bottle.

4. Shake mixture well to mix.

5. Apply using a cotton pad or cloth after you wash your face daily.

NOTE: Vitamin oxidizes quickly. So recipes should be made in little quantities.

Vitamin C Facial Serum

Works well for a drier skin.

Ingredients

   1/2 teaspoon natural Vitamin C Powder

   8 drops lavender essential oil, if desired.

   Food grade glycerin

Instructions

1. Mix vitamin C powder, glycerin and the essential oil.

2. Mix well until well combined.

3. Transfer ingredients into a dropper bottle, glass bottle or spray bottle.

4. Shake mixture well to mix.

5. Apply using a cotton pad or cloth after you wash your face daily.

NOTE: Vitamin oxidizes quickly. So recipes should be made in little quantities.

If you have really dry skin or don't want to use witch hazel, you can use food grade glycerin in place of the witch hazel. This will produce a serum instead of a toner. Either one should be made in small batches and often because Vitamin C oxidizes so quickly.

Aloe Vera Herbal Infusion Cleanser

This Aloe cleanser befits only royalty. It leaves your skin beautiful, soft and luxurious.

Ingredients

Makes: 1 (4 ounce) Jar

1/4 cup/5 tablespoons aloe vera gel

1 tablespoons castile soap

2 tablespoons sweet almond oil

20-60 drops Essential oils

Instructions

1. Pour aloe vera gel into a bottle; use a funnel.

2. Shake bottle to break aloe vera chunks up.

3. Measure in castile soap, sweet almond oil and essential oils into the bottle.

4. Vigorously shake the bottle until contents mixes well.

NOTE: Bottle content may separate if left for a while. Shake before use.

5. Apply by wetting your face with warm water; pour a small but rich dollop of cream on your clean palms.

6. Rub your palms together and start to apply on your forehead and work your way to your cheeks, nose and to your neck.

7. Close your pores by rinsing your face with cool water, using a muslin cloth.

8. Use an unused towel to pat your face dry.

NOTE: If you have dry skin, use 3 tbsps of sweet almond oil and skip the use of castile soap.

For the essential oils, if you have sensitive skin, use 20 drops. You can use any of these essential oils; they work well for these cleanser; lavender, carrot seed or tea tree essential oils.

Beautiful Face Cream Recipe

This recipe leaves your face beautifully rich and healthy. It has an out of this world smooth consistency and velvety feel that makes your skin soft and alive.

Ingredients

¼ cup organic Olive Oil or Calendula Herbal Oil

¼ cup organic Grapeseed Oil

¼ cup organic Sesame Oil

1/16 cup Beeswax pastilles

1/16 cup organic Coconut Oil

½ cup organic Aloe Vera Gel

1 cup organic Hydrosol of your choice

8-15 drops of any favorite essential oil

¼ teaspoon Vitamin E Oil

Instructions

1. Melt beeswax slowly in a stainless steel saucepan until liquefied.

2. In another stainless steel saucepan over very low heat, mix oils together and warm thoroughly.

3. Mix aloe gel and hydrosol in a small bowl.

4. Warm a double boiler, on low heat.

5. Set aside approx. 10 (2 ounce) glass jars with covers.

6. Transfer half of the warmed oil mixture into the top portion of the double boiler.

7. Measure in a quarter ounce of the melted beeswax into the double broiler.

8. Measure in 6 ounces of aloe gel and hydrosol mixture into a blender, with a quarter tsp of vit.E oil.

9. Measure in your favorite essential oils into the blender.

NOTE: For your essential oils, lavender, orange, rose, sandalwood or chamomile essential oils are great options.

10. Cover the blend and blend to combine, for about a minute.

11. Take out the cover's middle portion in your blender.

12. Set the blender to low and very carefully and slowly transfer the wax and warm oil mixture into the center of the "whirling" waters in the blender.

NOTE: It is very important that you are careful about this process. Patiently pour in a very slow thin stream. At first the cream will look very odd but will gradually reach a thick consistency and will be emulsified. At this point, the blender sound will change.

13. Put the blender off.

14. Use a small spoon or spatula to clean mixtures off the insides of the blender and its blades.

15. Mix cream thoroughly.

16. Put the blender on again and blend finally until a fine mixing consistency is reached.

17. Transfer cream into jars that have been set aside, using the spatula where necessary to get all the cream out.

18. Repeat process for second batch.

19. Store in a freezer for 2-3 hours. Label and Apply as necessary.

Homemade Dandy Facial Serum

Ingredients

½ cup aloe vera gel

1 tbsp dried dandelion leaves and flowers/5-6 fresh dandelion leaves and flowers

1 tsp vitamin E

Instructions

1. Mix dandelions and aloe gel into a blender or food processor.

2. Blend for 5 to 10 times and set aside for 30-60 minutes to steep.

3. Transfer mixture to a cloth strainer or mesh and strain the dandelions from the aloe vera gel.

NOTE: Make sure there are no dandelions remaining after straining. For best results, strain twice.

4. Measure in a tsp if vit. E oil into the mixture.

5. Store in container that is dark and that has a dropper as cover.

6. You can store in a bathroom drawer. It has a shelf life of 6 to 12 weeks.

7. Apply after using your toner and before using your moisturizer. Smooth 8 to 10 drops of this facial serum over your neck, décolleté and face. Allow to dry before moisturizing.

NOTE: Some certain number of people is sensitive to the latex milk found in dandelion. If you find any reaction like rashes on your skin, discontinue usage and tweak recipes, using only leaves.

Homemade Herbal tea Skin Clearing Face Mist

Ingredients

1 drop Tea tree oil

2 bags Peppermint tea bags

Pink Himalayan sea salt

1 drop Lavender essential oil

Instructions

1. Boil a cup of strong peppermint tea in a pot.

2. Stir in sea salt and stir to incorporate.

3. Measure in the tea tree oil into the mixture and stir well.

4. Stir in the lavender essential oil and set aside for a while, to cool.

5. Transfer mixture into a spray glass bottle.

Hibiscus face mask

Ingredients

¼ cup brown rice flour

Yogurt

1 heaping tsp hibiscus powder

Aloe vera gel

Instructions

1. In a mixing bowl, measure in hibiscus powder and rice flour together.

2. Transfer into a jar and cover well.

3. Before each use mix 2 tsps of the dry face mask powder with sufficient amount of aloe gel and yogurt till a paste like consistency is reached.

4. Rub a thick layer on your face and leave to dry for 10 to 15 minutes.

5. Wash your face with warm water after 10 to 15 minutes.

Five Minutes Homemade Herb Facial Steam

With summer time approaching, and the skin damages and the cold and nasal congestions of the winter lingering. You can go the old-school way and give yourself a treat with steam.

Ingredients

Few cups of water

Any of your favorite fresh herbs (rosemary, basil or mint)

Instructions

1. Wash your face,

2. Place few cups of water until it almost boils.

3. In a large bowl, pour in hot water, measure in a handful of rosemary, basil or mint.

4. Apply by bending over the bowl of fresh herbs and hot water, covering your head with a clean towel.

5. Do this until the steam dissipates or for five minutes.

NOTE: If you don't have access to rosemary, basil or mint, you can toss in peppermint, chamomile or lavender tea bags.

Homemade Caffeine Eye Serum

Having puffy eyes or dark circles when enough sleep hasn't been gotten is sometimes hereditary. It happens because oxygenated blood pools under the eyes. Your sleeping position can also be a major contributing factor to this condition.

Ingredients

1/2 cup ground coffee

1 tablespoon Avocado oil

Sweet almond oil

Serum bottle

Instructions

1. In a jar that can be well covered, combine ground coffee and sweet almond oil together.

2. Cover the jar well. Make sure it is airtight.

3. Set aside for a week to infuse oils.

4. Strain the oil from the coffee; using a mesh strainer or cheesecloth.

5. Transfer infused oil to another container or jar.

6. Measure in avocado into the oil content and stir until incorporated.

7. Transfer into a jar and cover.

8. Apply few minutes before bed, using your ring finger to apply on the skin area surrounding your eyes.

DIY Peeling Mask

Ingredients

A small jar

2 tbsps milk

1 packet unflavored gelatin

2 drops eucalyptus essential oil or grapefruit essential oil (or your favorite).

Instructions

1. Measure in a full packet of unflavored gelatin into a small mixing bowl.

2. Measure essential oil into the bowl.

3. Stir in the milk into the mixture in the mixing bowl.

NOTE: The mixture will become clumpy.

4. Place mixture in the microwave for 10 seconds.

NOTE: After you microwave mixture, it should not be clumpy, if it is still clumpy, microwave for 5 seconds more; stirring thoroughly.

5. Apply to your face fast, by slathering a finely thin layer on your face.

NOTE: Avoid your brows and your eyes.

6. Once the mask becomes dry on your face, wash it off and follow with it moisturizer.

DIY Anti Wrinkle Cream

Ingredients

2 teaspoons jojoba oil

3 teaspoons apricot kernel oil

1 teaspoon coconut oil

1 1/2 teaspoon beeswax pastilles

3 teaspoons Rosehip seed oil

6-10 teaspoons rose-water

Instructions

1. Combine jojoba oil, beeswax pastilles, coconut oil, rosehip seed oil and apricot kernel oil together.

2. Transfer into a double boiler to melt over medium low heat for approximately 5 to 8 minutes.

3. Stir to combine and set aside to cool for some minutes.

4. Transfer into an electric blender and blend. Measure rose water slowly and in a steady stream into the electric blender as you blend mixture.

5. Blend until a fluffy cream-like consistency is reached.

6. Refrigerate until you want to use.

NOTE: For a very oily skin, increase the rose water amount to 12-20 teaspoons.

Super Botox Facial Scrub

Ingredients:

   1 tbsp baking soda

   1 drop of pure lavender essential oil

   ½ tbsp honey

   1 drop pure frankincense essential oil

Instructions:

1. Mix honey and baking soda together until it is pasty.

2. Toss in frankincense and lavender oils.

3. Open up your pores by placing a warm towel over your face for a minute thereabout.

4. Apply by massaging your skin with facial scrub to your face gently for 3 to 5 minutes in circular motions.

NOTE: Your face may be slightly red for a while; this is because dead skin has been removed from your face.

5. Wash off and rinse with water that is warm.

NOTE: This facial scrub should be used not more than once or twice weekly. To balance your skin pH, it is important that you splash rose water on your face after steps 1-5.

Homemade Beard Oil Recipe

Ingredients

10-12 tbsps sweet almond oil or jojoba oil or apricot oil

2-3 drops tea tree essential oil

2-3 drops lavender essential oil

2-3 drops cedarwood essential oil

8 ounce dropper bottle

5 drops Vitamin E oil

Instructions

1. Combine sweet almond oil and the essential oils into dropper bottle

2. Measure in vitamin E oil.

3. Shake bottle vigorously to mix

4. Apply as needed.

Homemade Vitamin C Serum Toner Recipe

Ingredients

1/2 tsp natural real food Vitamin C Powder

2 tbsps vegetable glycerine

1 tsp distilled water

A dark colored container to store

Instructions

1. Combine vitamin C powder and water together to dissolve.

2. Measure in the vegetable glycerin.

3. Set aside in a refrigerator for 4 weeks or more.

4. Apply as a toner after you have cleansed

NOTE: Excess Vitamin C can burn the skin if it is highly concentrated. Adhere strictly to instructions; don't add more than specified amount.

Firming Eye Cream Recipe

For a sterling eye treatment, this recipe will help give your eyes that super treatment needed.

Ingredients

Makes: 4 ounces

   1/4 cup green tea

   1 tablespoon rosehip seed oil

   1/8 teaspoon NeoDefend

   1/4 teaspoon vitamin E

   1 tablespoon sweet almond oil

   1 drop carrot seed essential Oil

   1 teaspoon emulsifying wax

   3 drops lavender Essential Oil

Instructions

1. Fill 2 medium sized sauce pans half way with water.

2. On medium heat, place 1 glass bowl that has a spout into each sauce pan.

3. Measure in rosehip seed oil, wax, sweet almond oil and vit.E oil into one of the glass bowl inside the sauce pan.

TIP: Meanwhile before step 1, brew one cup of green tea

4. Measure in NeoDefend and the brewed green tea into the second glass bowl in the other sauce pan.

5. Heat the mixtures in the two separate sauce pans until the wax melts completely.

7. Take the temperatures of the two sauce pans with a thermometer.

NOTE: Both have to be at same for the cream to set when combined. Otherwise your cream would not set.

8. When both mixtures in the saucepan reach 130°F, pour the green tea mixture into the rosehip seed oil mixture.

9. Combine cream together, using a hand blender.

10. Mix every ten minutes thereabout for 30-60 minutes, until water doesn't separate at the bottom anymore

11. Measure in essential oils into the mixture once it is fully mixed.

12. This cream works well under make up, use morning and night.

Bentonite Clay and Charcoal Detoxifying Face Mask

Spray your face lightly with toner as the mask begins to dry to prevent red skin and irritation as the clay mask dries off.

Ingredients

4 capsules activated charcoal

½ cup bentonite clay

1 tbsp finely ground oatmeal

1 tbsp finely ground green tea

1 tbsp finely ground hibiscus

1 tbsp finely ground rosehips

Instructions

1. Mix all the powders in a wooden or glass bowl.

NOTE: This is very important; make you use utensils that are non metal. The Betonite clay has negative charges and it can be deactivated if metal utensils are used.

2. Mix thoroughly until finely mixed.

3. Keep in a cool, dry place and store in a plastic or glass jar.

4. Apply by mixing 1 to 2 tsps of the powdered detoxifying face mask with 2 to 4 tsps of hydrosol or water.

5. Set aside for five minutes before applying to your face.

6. Leave the mask on your face for 15 to 20 minutes.

NOTE: from time to time, spray your face with hydrosol, water or toner whenever your face feels tight, dry or itchy.

7. Use a wash cloth and rinse face off, exfoliating your skin gently in the process.

8. To lock in the moisture and close your pores, apply toner and moisturizer after rinsing.

CHAPTER TWO - ORGANIC SKIN AND BEAUTY RECIPES FOR THE LIPS (LIP BALM, SCRUBS, TREATMENT...)

Cold Sore Lip Balm

Ingredients

4 tbsps lemon balm infused oil

1/2 tbsp tamanu oil

1 1/2 tbsp of coconut oil

2 scant tbsps beeswax

1/2 tbsp castor oil

15 drops tea tree oil

1 tbsp mango butter/shea butter

2 drops of clove bud oil (if desired, for pain relief)

25 drops of peppermint essential oil

Instructions

1. In a container that can withstand high heat, mix beeswax, lemon balm infused oil, tamanu oil, coconut oil, castor oil, and shea butter/mango butter together.

2. Mix until thoroughly combined.

3. Fill a saucepan partway with water.

4. Transfer the heatproof container into the saucepan over medium low heat and heat.

5. Heat until the container mixture melts completely.

6. Take away from the heat and measure in the tea tree oil, clove bud oil, and peppermint essential oil

7. Transfer into glass jars.

8. Once lip balm sets, cover and keep away from the sun

9. Apply with cotton swabs and avoid dipping your hand twice at go into the lip balm to avoid contamination.

NOTE: This balm can also be used for patches of dry skin and minor scrapes.

Flavored Homemade Hippy Lippy Lip Balms

Ingredients

3 tablespoons coconut oil, unrefined

1 1/2 tablespoon beeswax pastilles

1 tablespoon mango butter

vitamin E (if desired)

1/2 tablespoon castor oil (if desired, for a glossy look)

Instructions

1. Combine beeswax and mango butter in a small bowl.

2. Transfer into a double boiler and melt.

3. Once beeswax mixture is melted, toss in the coconut oil into the beeswax mixture and melt.

4. Take off from heat.

5. If using, mix in castor oil, vitamin E, and essential oils, and mix well.

6. Transfer into clean and sterile containers.

7. Set aside to cool before use.

Chocolate Cocoa Lip Balm with Mint

This lip balm recipe is very sumptuous; it will be difficult to keep from licking your lips every now and then.

Ingredients

  3 tablespoon coconut oil, unrefined

  1 1/2 tablespoon beeswax pastilles

  1 tablespoon cocoa butter

  25 drops peppermint essential oil

  Vitamin E (if desired)

Instructions

1. Combine beeswax, chocolate chips and cocoa butter in a small bowl.

2. Transfer into a double boiler and melt.

3. Once beeswax mixture is melted, toss in the coconut oil into the beeswax mixture and melt.

4. Take off from heat.

5. If using, mix in vitamin E and peppermint essential oil, and mix well.

6. Transfer into clean and sterile containers.

7. Set aside to cool before use.

Peppermint Lavender Lip Balm

Ingredients

3 tablespoon coconut oil, unrefined

1 1/2 tablespoon beeswax pastilles

1 tablespoon organic unrefined shea butter

25 drops peppermint essential oil and lavender essential oil

Vitamin E (if desired)

Instructions

1. Combine beeswax and unrefined shea butter butter in a small bowl.

2. Transfer into a double boiler and melt.

3. Once beeswax mixture is melted, toss in the coconut oil into the beeswax mixture and melt.

4. Take off from heat.

5. If using, mix in vitamin E and essential oils, and mix well.

6. Transfer into clean and sterile containers.

7. Set aside to cool before use.

Cinnamint Spice Lip Plumping Lip Balm

Ingredients

3 tablespoons coconut oil, unrefined

1 tablespoon organic unrefined Shea butter

1 1/2 tablespoons beeswax pastilles

6 drops cinnamon leaf essential oil

10 drops peppermint essential oil

1-2 teaspoons beet root powder/alkanet root powder (if desired, for pink/red lip tint)

4 drops clove bud essential oil

Vitamin E (if desired)

Instructions

1. Combine beeswax and unrefined shea butter in a small bowl.

2. Transfer into a double boiler and melt.

3. Once beeswax mixture is melted, toss in the coconut oil into the beeswax mixture and melt.

4. Take off from heat.

5. If using, mix in alkanet root powder, vitamin E, and essential oils, and mix well.

6. Transfer into clean and sterile containers.

7. Set aside to cool before use.

Peppermint Rose Syrup Lip Balm

Ingredients

1 tbsp shea butter

1/2 tbsp castor oil

2 1/2 tbsps rose infused oil

Powdered alkanet root (for natural color)

1 tbsp beeswax

15-20 drops of peppermint essential oil

Instructions

For Lip Balm Color

1. In a small bowl, measure in few drops of rose infused oil and then mix in a very little amount of powdered alkanet root.

2. Stir to combine until a dark red thick consistency is reached. Put aside.

Making the Lip Balm

3. In another bowl, toss in beeswax, the oils remaining and shea butter.

4. Transfer shea butter mixture into a double boiler over medium low heat, and melt.

5. Take off the heat and mix in the alkanet/rose infused oil paste a little at a time until you reached the kind of color you desire.

NOTE: To get a pink color, use less of the alkanet paste, for more of red, use more of the paste.

6. Measure in the essential oil.

7. Transfer lip balm into tubes.

Homemade Chapped Lip Treatment, Honey Lip Balm and Scrub

Ingredients

1 tbsp shea butter

1 tsp almond oil

1 tsp honey

1 tsp beeswax, grated

1 tsp olive oil

3-4 drops vanilla extract

5 white chocolate chips

Lip balm container

Instructions

1. In a small bowl, mix olive oil and almond oil together.

2. Measure in the vanilla extract and mix together.

3. In a bowl that is microwave safe, melt the beeswax in short burst until almost melting completely.

4. Measure in the chocolate chips and continue to heat until both beeswax and chocolate chips are melted totally.

5. Combine the beeswax mixture with the oils in the bowl.

6. Combine until well incorporated.

7. Pour into a clean and sterile lip balm container and allow it set.

NOTE: You can refrigerate to speed up the rate of solidifying.

TIP: a) Rub a little coconut and a little honey to your lips over night to treat chapped lips.   b) With clean fingers, pierce a capsule of vitamin E and apply to cracks in the mouth.

Lavender Mint Natural Lip Balm

Ingredients

2 tablespoons coconut oil

2 tablespoons beeswax pastilles

2 tablespoons Shea butter

8 drops lavender essential oils

12 drops peppermint essential oils

Lip balm containers (tubes or metal tins)

Instructions

1. In a dry, clean and sterile mason jar, mix in beeswax, shea butter and coconut oil together.

2. Partly fill a pot with water and place on low heat.

3. Place mason jar into partly filled pot of water,

4. Melt beeswax mixture, stirring from time to time, for 10 minutes or until beeswax mixture melts completely.

5. Turn off the heat and set jar with water and pot aside to cool.

NOTE: Leave mixture in the water, with the heat turned off, so that beeswax mixture wouldn't solidify too fast.

7. Measure in essential oils to the melted beeswax mixture and stir thoroughly to incorporate.

8. Transfer contents into lip balm containers.

NOTE: If any leftover solidified as you were pouring into containers, reheat following the instructions above and transfer to other lip balm containers.

Sugar Lip Exfoliating Scrub

This recipe helps to remove dead skin peels from our lips, also helps to reveal the gentle skin beneath.

Ingredients

1 tbsp of white sugar/brown sugar

1 drop of vanilla (if desired)

1 tbsp of honey (or a little coconut oil/olive oil)

Instructions

1. Combine olive oil or coconut oil or honey with brown sugar together.

2. Mix thoroughly until well combined.

3. Transfer into a clean, dry and sterile container.

4. Apply 1-2 times weekly, vigorously rub the scrub on the lips to remove dead skin peels.

NOTE: Let scrub stay for a minute and rinse off with a washcloth that's damp.

5. Use lip balm after applying this scrub.

NOTE: Don't overuse recipe.

CHAPTER THREE - ORGANIC SKIN AND BEAUTY RECIPES FOR THE HANDS AND FEET

Peppermint Foot Balm Recipe

This recipe is the answer for tired feet after a long day's job in work boots, high heels, or even flips flops. It helps to soothe your heels, cracked and dry feet.

Ingredients

Makes: 1 cup

  1/4 cup olive oil infused with chamomile and calendula

  1/4 cup cocoa butter

  1/4 cup lavender infused coconut oil

  25 drops peppermint essential oil

  25g beeswax, grated

  5 drops vanilla essential oil

  10 drops lemongrass essential oil

  5 drops lavender essential oil

5 drops tea tree essential oil

Instructions

1. Combine grated beeswax, cocoa butter and oils together into a bowl.

2. Transfer into a double boiler over mid-low heat and melt.

NOTE: Don't leave oils to warm excessively.

3. Once double boiler mixture is melted, measure in essential oils and stir to incorporate.

4. Transfer into another container that can withstand heat.

5. Set aside to cool, for 6 to 8 hours.

6. Apply to feet after bathing or showering at night for the next two weeks.

Homemade Hand Cream

This recipe is a specialty for hands that are rough with hard work. We love to ride horses and we hold their reins, we have built one thing or the other, we knead dough and all, cleared bushes, shoveled manure, planted and weeded. So this recipe would be a great gift to your parents to help soften their hands that have been roughened by age.

Ingredients

1/4 cup shea butter

1 tbsp beeswax

1/8 cup sweet almond oil

10 drops cedarwood essential oil

10 drops myrrh essential oil

Instructions

1. In a double boiler, combine sweet almond oil, beeswax and shea butter together.

2. Stir to mix from time to time as it melts

3. Take off from heat and set aside 5 to 10 minutes.

4. Measure in the cedarwood and myrrh essential oil.

5. Transfer mixture into a glass container that us small and set aside for few hours to set.

6. Apply to dry hands as frequently as possible, after a long day's work or working with dirt.

Lavender Calendula Healing Hand Salve

Ingredients

3 oz. olive oil

1 tbsp lavender buds

2 oz. coconut oil

2 oz. beeswax pellets (white or yellow)

1 tbsp calendula petals, dried

2 oz. shea butter

Instructions

1. In a glass measuring cup, measure olive oil and coconut oil.

2. Place glass jar in a microwave and heat gently.

3. Measure in the lavender buds and dried calendula petals

4. Turn off the heat and set aside for 30 minutes to an hour and then strain.

NOTE: You should warm again if mixture is too thick to strain.

5. Pour the infused oil into the glass measuring cup and then measure in the beeswax.

6. Put mixture into a microwave and reheat.

7. Take out of the microwave and measure in the shea butter.

NOTE: The shea butter will melt fast, make sure you mix thoroughly.

8. Set aside to cool a little and toss in the lavender essential oil.

9. Transfer into a well covered container. Set aside to cool totally.

TIP: It will last for several months, should be used as frequently as you want.

Super Rich Herbal Foot Butter

Ingredients

1/2 cup (4 oz.) shea butter

4 1/2 tsps (3/4 oz.) beeswax, grated

2 tbsps (1 oz.) avocado oil

1 1/2 tsps non-GMO vitamin E oil

2 tbsps lanolin

30 drops your favorite essential oils

Instructions

1. Combine shea butter, lanolin, beeswax and avocado oil into a small mixing bowl.

2. Stir to combine until well mixed.

3. Transfer into a pot over low heat; heat until completely melted; stirring from time to time.

4. Take off from heat and measure in the essential oil(s) and vitamin E oil.

5. Stir mixture well to incorporate oils.

6. Transfer into a jar. Set aside to cool until mixture solidifies.

7. Apply by massaging a little amount into any part of your body or feet that needs revitalizing and uplifting.

Honey and Wild Rose Hand Cream

This cream evens your skin tone, reduces inflammation, and has a mildly astringent effect on open pores.

Ingredients

Makes: about 100ml

  1/3 cup (84ml) Rosewater

  1/2 teaspoon (2 grams) Sodium Lactate

  1/4 teaspoon (1.8 grams) Honey

  1/8 teaspoon (0.5 gram) Liquid Germall Plus

  1/4 + 1/8 teaspoon (1.5 grams) Geogard Ultra

NOTE: The last 2 ingredients are preservatives if you want to keep the lotion in the refrigerator for more than seven days, or at room temperature.

  1 teaspoon (5grams) Sunflower Oil

  1/4 teaspoon (1.3 grams) Rice Bran oil

  1/4 teaspoon (1.2 grams) Shea Butter

  2.5 teaspoon (3.8 grams) Emulsifying Wax

1/8 teaspoon (0.5 gram) Cocoa Butter

1/16 teaspoon (0.2 gram) Xanthan Gum

10-20 drops of (Rose Geranium essential oil, Rose essential oil, and/or (0.5-1 grams) Ylang Ylang essential oil, if desired.

20 drops (1 grams) Vitamin E Oil

Instructions

1. In a large mixing bowl, combine rosewater, sodium lactate, honey, liquid germall plus and geogard ultra together.

2. In another bowl, combine sunflower oil, rice bran oil, shea butter oil, emulsifying wax, cocoa butter, xathan gum, vitamin E oil and the essential oils together.

3. Transfer both contents into two separate mason jars.

4. In a saucepan with a dishcloth at the bottom. Place mason jars in the dishcloth lined sauce pan.

5. Pour water into the saucepan until the content level of the mason jar has been passed slightly.

NOTE: Do not use a microwave please.

6. Bring water filled saucepan to a simmer, and continue simmering for 20 minutes.

NOTE: Both Mason jar contents must be at 176°F temperature.

7. Take out the mason jars carefully trying not to scald your fingers.

8. Slowly and gently transfer the oil jar mixture into the rosewater jar mixture and keep stirring using a spoon.

9. After the oil jar mixture has been completely emptied, use a mini whisk to whisk the whole mixture together for some minutes until a milk creamy consistency is reached.

10. Set cream aside to cool well.

11. Measure in the essential oils and vitamin E oil into the cream mixture and mix to incorporate.

12. Transfer hand lotion into plastic or glass jar and allow the cream to set.

Hand Salve for Men

Ingredients

1/2 cup calendula, dried

1 cup sweet almond oil/olive oil/apricot kernel oil/sunflower oil

1/8 cup comfrey, dried

7/10 ounce herbal infused oil

1/2 cup avocado oil (if desired)

7/10 ounce beeswax

7/10 ounce coconut oil

7 drops cedarwood essential oil (if desired)

11 drops bay essential oil (if desired, or any of your favorite essential oil)

4 drops lemon balm essential oil (if desired)

Instructions

To make the infusion

1. In a small jar, mix herbs and oils until the jar is filled to the brim.

2. Cover the jar well.

3. Set aside for 2 weeks or a month to infuse oils.

TIP: On the flip side; use warm water bath for an hour or two hours to infuse the oils.

To make the salve

1. Use a cheesecloth or coffee filter to strain the oil from the herbs.

2. In a double boil, mix beeswax, coconut oil and infused oil together.

3. Melt the mixture totally and set aside for some minutes.

NOTE: Make sure you don't allow the mixture solidify. Mix well to combine.

4. Measure in the essential oils.

5. Mix well and pour into the glass container. Cover well.

This recipe will stay up to 6 to 12 months or even more.

6. Apply to cracked, work worn and dried hands.

DIY Cuticle Cream

This homemade recipe is good for a quality nail care routine, it's a good way to pamper your fingernails.

Ingredients

1 tablespoon organic beeswax

5 drops of lavender essential oil*

2 tablespoons organic shea butter

2-4 drops of Vitamin E oil

5 drops of orange essential oil*

Instructions

1. In a mason jar, mix shea butter and beeswax together.

2. Fill 1/3 of a small saucepan partly with water and bring to boiling.

3. Place mason jar into the saucepan with boiling water.

4. Melt beeswax mixture; remove the jar from the water carefully.

5. Measure in the vitamin E oil and essential oils and stir to incorporate.

6. Pour mixture into a small jar, container or canister.

7. Set aside to cool completely and allow to harden.

NOTE: Recipe can stay up to a year or more and doesn't need to be stored in a freezer.

You can skip essential oils in the ingredients if they are not handy.

8. Apply to the skin surrounding the nails and cuticles every night, before going to bed.

Rose & Kaolin Clay Foot Mask Recipe

Ingredients

Makes: 1 (8 ounce) jar

8 ounce glycerin liquid

2 mL vitamin E oil

3 mL avocado extract

2.4 mL optiphen ND

1 1/2 mL peppermint essential oil

1 cup Rose Clay

1 cup Kaolin Clay

Instructions

1. Combine kaolin clay and rose clay in a large mixing bowl.

2. Whisk bowl's content and set aside.

3. Mix avocado extract, glycerin liquid, peppermint essential oil, optiphen ND and vitamin E oil into another bowl.

4. Mix well to combine.

5. Stir in the liquid mixture into the clay mixture slowly.

6. Continue to stir until a fine consistency is reached.

NOTE: Eliminate all clumps.

7. Transfer mask into an 8 ounce bail jar.

8. Keep in a dry and cool place.

Lavender Mint Soothing Body Butter Foot Cream

Ingredients

1/4 cup extra virgin coconut oil

2 tablespoons calendula petals, dried

3/4 cup unrefined (Grade A) shea butter

8 drops lavender essential oil

2 tablespoons marshmallow root, dried (already cut up)

8 drops peppermint essential oil

Instructions

1. Preheat oven to 200°F.

2. Turn heat off. Melt shea butter and coconut oil in an oven safe pan on low heat.

3. Toss herbs in, mix until well combined and then place in the oven.

4. Leave herbs for 4 hours or more to steep.

5. Using cheesecloth or mesh strainer, strain herbs from oil; transfer infused oil into a small bowl that you will be using to whip the cream.

NOTE: Warm herb mixture on the stove incase the mixture hardens while in the oven, before straining.

6. Refrigerate oil for a few hours, until it becomes firm but not solid.

7. Take oil out of the refrigerator, and whip oil for half a minute, using a mixer.

NOTE: Use a spatula to mix any part of oil that is stuck at the bottom of the bowl.

8. Measure in essential oils and whip once more, for a minute.

NOTE: At this point, the whipped cream mixture will turn white peaks will be formed; it will look deliciously attractive and tempting to eat. Do not try to taste.

9. Transfer mixture into a clean jar.

10. Soak your feet for a while before bed time, and then apply this foot cream by rubbing it in very well at least 30 minutes before going to bed.

CHAPTER FOUR - ORGANIC SKIN AND BEAUTY RECIPES FOR THE BODY, (BATHS, BODY WASH, BODY BUTTER, SUNSCREENS, SCRUBS, LOTIONS...)

DIY Lotion Bars

Ingredients

3 oz. beeswax

20-40 drops of essential oil (if using, peppermint, orange, rose or lavender are great)

1 1/2 oz. shea butter

1 1/2 oz. cocoa butter

3 oz. calendula or any herbal infused oil

Instructions

1. Melt shea butter, cocoa butter and beeswax in a double boiler or a salve-making saucepan on lowest heat you can get.

NOTE: Stir often to keep from burning shea butter mixture.

2. After melting, add calendula oil or any other herbal infused oils.

NOTE: At this point, mixture may start to thicken slightly.

3. Continue to stir while on low heat until the mixture melts totally.

NOTE: It is important to set heat to low to avoid oils from going rancid from too much heat.

4. After you have melted the mixture completely, measure in the essential oils, if using.

5. Transfer mixture into flat sided tin containers or molds.

NOTE: If your environment happens to be as hot as mine, I suggest you use tin, to allow the lotion bars slip out easily.

6. Set aside to cool, until mixture hardens completely.

7. Pop lotion bars out from the tin or molds and use.

8. Store lotion bars in a cool, dry place.

NOTE: If they are in a very hot place, lotion bars will melt.

TIP: In case you can't get an herbal infused oil like calendula, you can make use of

3 oz. Grape seed or jojoba oil (or any other cosmetic oil that is easily absorbed by the skin)

Baby Bump Belly Balm Bar

Ingredients

Makes: approx. 2/3 cup

2 tbsps beeswax

5 tbsps cocoa butter

1/2 tbsp carnauba Wax

1 tbsp macadamia nut oil

1 tbsp hemp seed oil

1 tbsp meadowfoam seed oil

1 tbsp baobab oil

1 tbsp pomegranate seed oil

1 tbsp argan oil

1/2 tbsp vitamin E oil

Instructions

1. Combine carnuba wax, beeswax, cocoa butter, macadamia nut oil, hemp seed oil, meadowfoam seed oil and baobab oil together into a large mixing bowl.

2. Transfer mixture into a double boiler and melt mixture until fully melted; stirring occasionally.

3. Measure in vitamin E oil, pomegranate seed oil and argan oil into the mixture. Stir to melt and incorporate into the mixture.

4. Take mixture away from heat.

5. Transfer mixture into silicone molds.

6. Set molds aside to cool until the mixture solidifies.

Plantain Salve Recipe

Plantain is known for its great healing characteristics. It is used to treat skin irritations, wounds, cuts and scrapes, bug bites and many other skin problems.

Ingredients

Makes: 1/2 cup of salve.

   1/2 cup Olive oil

   1/2 oz. beeswax

   1/3 cup dried plantain

Instructions

1. Measure dried plantain and olive oil together.

2. Transfer into a well covered jar and set aside for 2 weeks to infuse the oil.

TIP: a) For an equally great and quicker oil infusion; Place herbs and oils in a very heavy saucepan over very low heat. b) Warm for 1/2 hour. The downside of this other approach is that the integrity of the herbs is compromised a little because of the heat. c) Turn heat off and set covered saucepan aside. This assures us a certain level of effectiveness.

3. Using a mesh strainer or cheesecloth, strain out all the oil from herbs.

4. In a heavy duty saucepan, measure beeswax and melt over very low heat.

5. Once saucepan content begins to melt, pour in the infused oil. Stirring until incorporated.

6. After melting beeswax totally. Transfer mixture into a clean and sterile jar.

7. Set aside to cool before you cover.

NOTE: This recipe will stay up to year.

Lavender Chamomile Body Lotion

No greasy after-feel; soothes dry skin and is well absorbed into the skin.

Ingredients

3 tbsps dried chamomile flowers

Almond, olive or grapeseed oil

3 tbsps dried lavender blossoms

2 tbsp beeswax, grated

1/2 cup water

1/8 tsp borax

Lavender tea

10 drops chamomile or lavender essential oils

Instructions

1. Combine almond oil with 1 tbsp of dried lavender blossoms and dried chamomile flowers into a jar with a good cover.

2. Cover well and set aside for 4 weeks to infuse oils.

NOTE: For best results, keep jar where the sun light can reach.

3. Once oils have been infused, use cheesecloth or mesh strainer to strain the flowers from the oil. Squeezing out every little bit of oil from the flower.

4. Bring water in a pot to boiling. Take off from heat after boiling and add the dried lavender blossoms remaining.

5. Lock the pot's lid in place and allow the flavor of the lavender blossoms to be released completely to make lavender tea.

6. Using cheesecloth or mesh strainer, strain the dried lavender blossoms from the water.

7. Combine beeswax and 1/2 cup of infused oil into a double boiler over medium low heat.

8. Heat until the mixture is completely melted.

9. Transfer strained lavender tea into a small pot and bring to boiling.

10. Measure borax into a bowl that can withstand heat and carefully pour in the lavender tea in; stir until borax dissolves completely.

11. In a blender or food processor, whip beeswax/oil mixture.

12. In a careful, steady and gentle stream, pour the borax/lavender tea mixture into the beeswax/oil mixture and continue to mix until the lotion emulsifies completely.

NOTE: Use a spoon to scrape the sides of the food processor from time to time.

13. Measure in the essential oils into the whipped mixture.

Sugar Scrub with Green Tea

It reduces the appearance of skin cellulites.

Ingredients

1 cup of coconut oil or grapeseed, olive oils

1 ½ cup of brown sugar

2 green tea bags

2 tsps of green tea powder

Instructions

1. Boil tea with distilled water, to make one hot green tea cup.

2. Leave aside to cool.

3. In a large bowl, measure in brown sugar, green tea powder and any of the oils in the ingredients, and mix together.

4. Measure in a little amount of the hot cup of green tea into the mixture per time and stir.

NOTE: Repeat step 4 as many times as possible until scrub mixture looks like wet sand from a beach side or grits.

Nourishing Homemade Body Wash

An extremely luxurious and gentle homemade body wash just for the beauty of your skin.

Ingredients

1/2 cup coconut milk canned, unsweetened

3 tsp vitamin E oil

2/3 cup castile soap

2 teaspoons vegetable glycerin, if desired

5 drops lavender essential oil

Instructions

1. Mix full-fat unsweetened coconut milk, vitamin E oil, castile soap, lavender essential oil and vegetable glycerin, if using.

2. Mix mixture together until well combined.

3. Transfer into a bottle or jar.

4. Keep refrigerated.

5. Shake well before application.

6. Pour a little on your washcloth and apply.

NOTE: Recipe doesn't have any preservative, and wouldn't stay more than a week due to the coconut milk contained in the recipe. You can substitute olive oil, almond oil or jojoba oil for the vegetable glycerin in the ingredient. When applying, you should be quick because of the coconut milk contained in the recipe.

Homemade Activated Charcoal Black Salve

This recipe is applied directly to sting and bug bite marks or splinter area on the skin.

Ingredients

1/4 cup calendula-infused oil

2 tsps beeswax pellets

1/4 cup coconut oil

3 tsps betonite clay

3 tsps (approx. 15 capsules) activated charcoal

10 drops tea tree essential oil

10 drops lavender essential oil

Instructions

1. Combine coconut oil and beeswax in a small bowl.

2. Mix well.

3. Transfer mixture into a double boiler and melt over medium low heat.

4. Once mixture has melted, measure in the calendular infused oil, betonite clay, activated charcoal, stirring to incorporate.

5. Remove from heat, and set aside to cool.

6. Measure in the essential oils; stirring to combine.

7. Transfer into a well covered glass jar. Store in a dark, cool and dry place.

8. Apply directly on affected skin area every 12 hours until affected skin is corrected.

Dry Winter Skin Body Butter

Ingredients

5 ounce of raw shea butter

4 tbsps solid coconut oil

2 tbsps avocado oil, almond oil, or grapeseed oil

Grapefruit, lavender, frankincense or ylang ylang essential oils

Instructions

1. Combine coconut oil and shea butter in a small bowl.

2. Mix with a mixer and combine thoroughly.

3. Once mixed; measure in avocado oil slowly and keep mixing until well incorporated.

4. Measure in the essential oil(s)

5. Stir to incorporate.

6. Transfer into a clean jar and refrigerate.

Homemade Suncream Herbal Treat

Ingredients

4 tbsps organic calendula infused oil

4 tbsps neem oil, organic

4 tbsps Aloe Vera Gel

4 tbsps coconut oil

4 tbsps sesame oil

4 tbsps Cocoa Butter or 10 wafers

4 tbsps Beeswax Pastilles

20 drops organic Lavender essential oil

4 tbsps organic Shea Butter

6 ounce containers

Instructions

1. Combine coconut oil, shea butter, cocoa butter and beeswax together in a small bowl.

2. Transfer into a double boiler and melt at medium low heat.

3. After double boiler content is melted, measure in the aloe gel and the oils.

4. Stir until everything blends well. Take off the heat.

5. Measure in vitamin E oil and the essential oils.

6. Stir until well incorporated.

7. Transfer mixture into the prepared containers and set aside to cool before locking cover in place.

NOTE: Wait for an hour before use or over the night preferably.

8. Apply before going out into the sun.

DIY (Cloth-Diaper-Safe) Diaper Balm

Ingredients

1 oz. olive oil

1 oz. coconut oil

2 tsps dried chamomile flowers

1 oz. cocoa butter, chopped

1 oz. shea butter

5 drops Tea Tree essential oil

½ oz. beeswax, chopped

2-3 drops Eucalyptus essential oil

2-3 drops Lavender essential oil

2-3 Grapefruit essential oil

2-3 drops Sweet Orange essential oil

Instructions

1. In a small saucepan over low heat, heat olive oil for approx. 10 minutes.

NOTE: Do not bring olive oil to boiling.

2. Toss in the dried chamomile flowers, cook and keep stirring for 10 additional minutes.

3. Remove saucepan from the heat, and set aside for flavors to be released for 1-2 hours.

4. Using a mesh strainer or cheesecloth, strain the chamomile from the oil.

5. Transfer strained oil into a double boiler and measure in shea butter, coconut oil, beeswax and cocoa butter.

6. Melt shea butter mixture until completely melted.

7. Take off from heat and transfer mixture into a bowl.

8. Set mixture aside till it cools.

9. Measure in tea tree, eucalyptus, lavender, grapefruit and sweet orange essential oils. Stir to combine well.

10. Mix mixture on high with a stick blender or stand mixer until the mixture changes from a clear liquid to a whitish solid form.

NOTE: IF in time, this change doesn't occur, or mixture is too watery; refrigerate mixture for 5 to 10 minutes.

11. Scrape bowl sides with a spoon and repeat mixing process.

NOTE: If repeating process doesn't work, measure in more cocoa butter or beeswax until desired thickness is attained.

12. Transfer by scooping into a jar and cover well.

13. Keep in cool, dry place. Do not use for more than 1 year.

Homemade Body Scrub with Coffee

This recipe keeps your skin soft, hydrated and moisturized.

Ingredients

Makes: 4-5 (4 ounce) Jelly jars.

 1 cup coconut oil

 1/3 cup fresh coffee grounds

 ½ cup sugar

 4-5 (4 ounce) jelly jars

 2-3 tablespoons olive oil

Instructions

1. Toss in sugar, coconut oil, olive oil and coffee grounds into a medium fairly large bowl.

2. Stir to combine and mix well until thoroughly combined.

3. Transfer mixture into clean and sterile jelly jars, cover well; label.

4. Store in a cool, dry place.

Homemade Shaving Cream

This shaving cream makes your skin luxuriantly pampered with this recipe. It's a great alternative for those with skins that are sensitive.

Ingredients

4 tablespoons solid shea butter

3 tablespoons coconut oil

2 tablespoons sweet almond oil

10-12 drops pure lavender essential oil, if desired

Instructions

1. Mix coconut oil and shea butter together

2. Transfer into a double boiler over very low heat and melt.

3. Stir from time to time. Take mixture off heat once mixture has melts totally.

4. Measure in lavender oil and almond and stir to incorporate oils well.

5. Pour mixture into a bowl and refrigerate to allow mixture solidify.

6. Whip shaving cream mixture using an electric mixer or a stand mixer.

7. Set whipped mixture aside before you transfer in a well covered jar or container.

TIP: Do not use beyond a month.

Lavender Oatmeal Tub Tea

Ingredients

Makes: approx. 9 teabags

2 cups Epsom salts

15-20 drops lavender essential oil

2 full tbsp lavender, dried

1 cup powdered milk

1 cup oatmeal

Instructions

1. In a large mixing bowl, combine lavender essential oil, dried lavender and Epsom salts together.

2. Mix in powdered milk into the mixing bowl mixture.

3. Use a blender or food processor, grind oatmeal to coarse powder.

4. Measure in ground oatmeal into mixing bowl.

5. Stir to combine mixing bowl mixture until well mixed.

6. Using a spoon, transfer mixture into 9 Jumbo-sized (size 4) tea filters.

7. Fold teabags at the top a few times and string tea bags.

8. Apply, one tea bag to a warm bath.

Deliciously scented Homemade Grapefruit Scrub

This out of this world grapefruit scrub leaves your skin with a beautiful and sweet fragrance. It moisturizes your skin and leaves it silky smooth.

Ingredients

Makes: 4-5 (4 ounce) Jelly jars

   1 cup coconut oil

3-4 tablespoons grapefruit juice

½ cup sugar

4-5 (4 ounce) Jelly jars

3 tablespoons grapefruit zest, if desired

Instructions

1. Grate grapefruit zest, using a grater.

2. Mix coconut oil, zest, grapefruit juice and sugar in a medium-sized mixing bowl.

3. Stir to combine mixing bowl mixture until well combined.

4. Transfer mixture into the jars.

5. Cover and label jars.

6. Store in a well covered jar and in a cool, dry place.

NOTE: Stir if any separation occurs before use. It will stay approximately half a year.

DIY Shaving Cream

Ingredients

Makes: 2 cups

1/2 (4 ounce) cup of coconut oil

1/4 cup olive oil

1/2 (4 ounce) cup shea butter

20-25 drops eucalyptus essential oil

Instructions

1. Combine shea butter and coconut oil in a mixing bowl.

2. Transfer bowl mixture into a double boiler over medium low heat and melt.

3. Once melted, take off from heat and transfer to a bowl.

4. Measure olive oil into the mixture and stir to incorporate.

5. Refrigerate until mixture solidifies.

6. Remove from the refrigerator.

7. Using a hand mixer or standing mixer, whip bowl's mixture until stiff peaks are formed, for 3 minutes.

8. Meanwhile, as you whip mixture, measure in the essential oils.

9. Transfer whipped shaving cream into a well covered jar and store.

Natural Homemade Blemish/Spot Eraser

This Blemish eraser treatment is super concentrated and should be applied to spots and blemishes directly, and not your entire body or face.

Ingredients

½ tsp organic tea tree oil

5 ml glass roller bottle

4 drops lavender essential oil

½ tsp organic tamanu oil

Instructions

1. In a glass bottle, combine tea tree oil, lavender essential oil and tamanu oil together.

2. Shake to combine glass bottle mixture.

3. Apply glass roller bottle mixture to the affected skin area.

NOTE: If applied to the face to get rid of spots and blemishes; few minutes after application, wash face and apply face oil or moisturizer.

Natural Homemade Rosemary Lavender Body Scrub

Preparation Time: 2 minutes

Total Time: 2 minutes

Ingredients

Makes: 1 pint-sized salt scrub jar.

2 cups Epsom salt

10-15 drops Lavender essential oil

1 cup organic extra-virgin coconut oil

Sprig of fresh rosemary, if desired

Instructions

1. Combine Epsom salt, lavender essential oil, rosemary and coconut oil into a large bowl.

2. Stir to combine well.

3. Pour into a mason jar and lock the cover in place.

Lavender and Honey Night Cream

Ingredients

  1/4 cup olive oil

  1 tablespoon Argan oil

  1 1/2 teaspoon raw honey

  1/2 teaspoon vitamin E oil

  1 teaspoon beeswax

  5 drops frankincense

  5 drops lavender essential oil

  4 ounce mason jar.

Instructions

1. Get a bowl that can withstand heat,

2. Toss in tiny pieces of beeswax and argan oil together in the bowl.

3. Heat until melted, as you stir frequently.

4. Set aside to cool for 2 to 3 minutes.

5. Mix in frankincense, lavender and vitamin E into the beeswax bowl.

6. Pour mixture into jar and cover well.

7. Store in a cool, dry place. Cream would stay 3 to 4 months.

NOTE: If due to extreme temperatures it liquefies, just refrigerate for a while.

8. Place 2 of your fingers on top of the cream and then apply to skin area.

CHAPTER FIVE - ORGANIC SKIN AND BEAUTY ANTI AGING & SKIN FIRMING RECIPES

It is possible to defy natural laws on aging. It is also possible to use natural, organic and homemade treatment to firm that skin up and look beautifully younger without visiting a plastic surgeon and using expensive cosmetics that go a long way to damage the body than help out.

Cypress Anti Aging and Firming Skin Serum

This serum is quick, easy and a great recipe that will firm your skin, moisturize and add that needed glow to your skin.

Ingredients

2 tablespoons Rosehip Seed Oil

10 drops of Cypress essential oil

2 tablespoons Sweet Almond Oil

7 drops of Frankincense Essential Oil

10 drops of Geranium essential oil

2 oz glass bottle

Instructions

1. Combine rosehip seed oil, cypress essential oil, sweet almond oil, frankincense essential oil and geranium essential oil together.

2. Transfer mixture into the glass bottle.

3. Shake well to combine well.

4. Apply once or twice daily.

NOTE: Less is more, apply a little at a time, just to cover your neck and face.

Honey/Avocado Moisturizer

Ingredients

3 tbsps of fresh cream

1 tbsp honey

1/4 avocado

Instructions

1. In an electric blender, combine avocado, honey and fresh cream.

2. Blend the contents of the blender until a smooth consistency is reached.

3. Rub on the skin and allow drying for 1 hour before washing off with water.

Wrinkle Eliminating Salad

The ingredients in this recipe have antioxidant properties that keep the skin from being damaged by the sun and help the blood circulate well. This ensures that the nutrient the skin needs is adequately circulated. Recipe is to be eaten.

Ingredients

   1/2 cup fresh blueberries

   1 kiwi, peeled and chopped

   1/2 cup strawberries

   1/2 cup organic orange juice

   1/2 cup pomegranate seeds

1 handful walnuts, chopped

Instructions

1. In a small bowl, combine blueberries, chopped kiwi, strawberries, and pomegranate seeds together.

2. Toss orange juice over blueberries mixture.

3. Sprinkle salad with walnuts. Serve, eat and enjoy

Anti Aging Toner with Basil

Ingredients

1 cup water

3 tbsps dried basil leaves

Instructions

1. Bring water to boiling in a pot

2. Toss crushed dried basil leaves into the hot water.

3. Using cheesecloth, strain water from the leaves.

4. Transfer into a spray bottle and apply to your skin.

NOTE: Make sure the toner is circulated on your face, using a cotton pad or ball.

Do this once a daily before cleansing your face.

Agave/Lemon Age Spot Fighter Scrub

Ingredients

1/2 cup rice, cooked

1 tbsp lemon juice

1 tbsp agave nectar

Instructions

1. Combine cooked rice, lemon juice and agave nectar together.

2. Blend together.

3. Apply a little scrub to your palm; make sure your palms are dry.

4. Use your other finger to move the scrub around in your palm in circular motions.

5. Rub this rice scrubs on callused hands and palms to soften.

NOTE: Rub firmly for 1-2 minutes with gentle pressure.

Sugar/Almond Anti Aging Facial Scrub

Ingredients

3 tbsps fresh cream

1/2 cup brown sugar

1 cup white sugar

2 tbsps olive oil

1/2 cup ground almonds

Instructions

1. Combine, fresh cream, brown sugar, white sugar, olive oil and ground almonds in a small mixing bowl.

2. Mix until well combined.

3. Use your hands while applying to your face in a circular motion.

4. Using warm water, rinse your face off

5. Transfer remaining recipe into a mason jar and keep refrigerated.

Anti Aging Coconut Deep Conditioner

Ingredients

1/2 cup mayonnaise

1 tsp coconut extract

1 tbsp coconut oil

Instructions

1. Combine all the ingredients into a small bowl.

2. Stir to combine well.

3. Apply deep conditioner on hair and cover your scalp.

NOTE: Any plastic wrap would do.

4. Allow to stay on for 20-30 minutes.

5. Rinse hair with water.

NOTE: Apply once a week.

Anti Aging Lip Exfoliator

Ingredients

   1/2 tsp moisturizing lotion

   1/4 tsp Kosher salt

   1/4 tsp fresh coffee grounds

Instructions

1. Combine moisturizing lotion, kosher salt and coffee grounds in a small bowl.

2. Rub on your mouth area completely and massage mouth area for 5 minutes.

3. Wipe your mouth clean with a wet and warm towel or wash cloth.

Rice Milk Cleanser

This recipe is known for its popularity among Japanese elites and royalty. It helps to smoothen your skin and exfoliate it.

Ingredients

2–3 tablespoons unsweetened organic rice milk

¼ cup brown rice flour (or rice bran flour)

Instructions

1. Combine rice milk and rice flour together.

2. Stir together until a fine paste consistency is reached.

3. Apply by massaging the cleanser on your skin.

NOTE: Application, should be tender and in circles.

4. Rinse with warm water and apply toner and moisturizer.

Cucumber Aloe Cold Anti Aging Cream

As you grow older, your skin dulls and dries simultaneously. This cream will help bring life and rejuvenate your skin once again; brightening your skin and returning the glory of your youth.

Ingredients

½ cup plain organic Greek yogurt

¼ cup peeled and chopped aloe flesh

¼ cup seeded and chopped cucumber

½ (juiced) lemon

Instructions

1. Combine yogurt, aloe flesh, cucumber and lemon together in a mixing bowl.

2. Blend bowl's content together in a food processor or electric blender.

3. Pulse until a smooth consistency is reached.

4. Place a mesh strainer lined with some layers cheese cloth over a bowl, then strain blenders content.

5. Strain over the night, covered.

6. In another bowl, pour the cream.

7. Apply cream generously to your face and let be for 30 minutes.

8. Wash off with a wet washcloth and apply toner.

TIP: On the flip side, the strained liquid remaining can be mixed with almond meal/rice flour, for a very effective face scrub.

Blueberry Granola Anti Aging Exfoliating Mask

Ingredients

¼ cup fresh organic blueberries

¼ cup raw almonds

2 tablespoons whole oats

1 tablespoon honey

1 tablespoon whole organic milk

Instructions

1. Mix blueberries, whole oats, almonds, organic milk and honey together into a small bowl.

2. Transfer bowl mixture into food processor or an electric blender.

3. Blend until a fine consistency is reached.

NOTE: While blending, you can add more milk, for required consistency.

4. Moisten your skin, and then apply richly to the skin.

5. Leave for 20 minutes to dry.

6. Rinse with warm water and apply your toner.

Anti Aging Walnut Blackberry Scrub

Ingredients

½ cup fresh organic blackberries

½ cup walnuts

Instructions

1. Place all ingredients together in a small bowl.

2. Transfer bowl mixture into a food processor or electric blender.

3. Blend until a smooth consistency is reached.

4. Moisten your skin, and then apply paste richly to the skin.

5. Massage skin area in circular motions.

6. Rinse with warm water and apply your toner and cleanser.

NOTE: If you don't have blackberries around, you can use black raspberries as a substitute.

Avocado Wheatgrass Anti Aging Mask

This anti aging recipe helps to renew the texture of the skin and also fights damage from aging-causing free radicals.

Ingredients

½ ripe avocado

1 tablespoon wheatgrass juice

2 tablespoon plain organic Greek yogurt

Instructions

1. Place all ingredients together in a small bowl.

2. Transfer bowl mixture into a food processor or electric blender.

3. Blend until a smooth consistency is reached.

4. Moisten your skin, and then apply paste richly to your skin.

5. Leave for 15 to 20 minutes to dry.

6. Rinse with warm water and apply your toner.

Apple Chia Honey Anti Aging Scrub

Ingredients

½ cup raw green apple, chopped

2 tablespoons chia seeds

2 tablespoons honey

Instructions

1. Place all ingredients together in a small bowl.

2. Transfer bowl mixture into a food processor or electric blender.

3. Blend until a smooth consistency is reached.

NOTE: Add water where necessary.

4. Set aside for 5 minutes.

5. Moisten your skin, and then apply paste richly to your skin.

6. Massage skin area in gentle and not too fast circular motions.

7. Rinse with warm water and apply your toner.

Coconut Avocado Anti Aging Body Oil

Ingredients

¼ cup avocado oil

¼ cup melted virgin coconut oil

¼ cup sweet almond oil

8 oz. bottle

Instructions

1. Place all ingredients together in a small bottle.

2. Shake vigorously to combine.

3. Rub on the body every day, from your shoulders to your toes.

4. Massaging the oils in.

Anti Aging Eye Roll On

Ingredients

1 tablespoon meadowfoam seed oil

1 1/2 teaspoon beeswax

2 teaspoons unrefined organic coconut oil

1/2 teaspoon Vitamin E oil

1/2 teaspoon shea butter

5 drops frankincense essential oil

4 drops carrot seed essential oil

8 drops lavender essential oil

Instructions

1. In a double boiler over low heat, measure coconut oil, meadowfoam seed oil, shea butter and beeswax in.

2. Take off from heat once sheabutter mixture melts completely.

3. Measure in vitamin E oil, frankincense, carrot seed and lavender essential oils into the mixture.

4. Transfer into a lip balm tube.

Firming Eye Cream Anti Aging Recipe

Ingredients

Makes: 4 ounces

   1/4 cup green tea

   1 tablespoon rosehip seed oil

   1/8 teaspoon NeoDefend

   1/4 teaspoon vitamin E

   1 tablespoon sweet almond oil

   1 drop carrot Seed essential Oil

   1 teaspoon emulsifying wax

   3 drops lavender Essential Oil

Instructions

1. Fill 2 medium sized sauce pans half way with water.

2. On medium heat, place 1 glass bowl that has a spout into each sauce pan.

3. Measure in rosehip seed oil, wax, sweet almond oil and vit.E oil into one of the glass bowl inside the sauce pan.

TIP: Meanwhile before step 1, brew one cup of green tea

4. Measure in NeoDefend and the brewed green tea into the second glass bowl in the other sauce pan.

5. Heat the mixtures in the two separate sauce pans until the wax melts completely.

7. Take the temperatures of the two sauce pans with a thermometer.

NOTE: Both have to be at same for the cream to set when combined. Otherwise your cream would not set.

8. When both mixtures in the saucepan reach 130°F, pour the green tea mixture into the rosehip seed oil mixture.

9. Combine cream together, using a hand blender.

10. Mix every ten minutes thereabout for 30-60 minutes, until water doesn't separate at the bottom anymore

11. Measure in essential oils into the mixture once it is fully mixed.

12. This cream works well under make up, use morning and night.

Natural Anti Aging Eye Cream

This recipe helps to restore youth, remove wrinkles and lines.

Ingredients

1/2 cup Organic coconut oil

10 drops frankincense essential Oil

6-8 Vitamin E capsules

Instructions

1. Place a saucepan over low heat.

2. Measure in coconut oil into the saucepan and melt for some minutes until completely melted.

3. Transfer melted coconut oil into a clean container with cover.

4. Pierce the vitamin E capsules and squeeze oil into the coconut oil container.

5. Stir to incorporate.

6. Measure in the essential oil.

7. Refrigerate for 30-60 minutes until the mixture solidifies.

NOTE: Once it solidifies, you don't need to refrigerate anymore.

8. Dap a little quantity of cream beneath your eyes at once at night and occasionally in the morning.

Homemade Anti-Aging Face Cream

Ingredients

Makes: approx. ½ cup

   ¼ cup almond oil

   2 tbsps beeswax

   2 tbsps coconut oil

   1 tbsp shea butter

   ½ tsp vitamin E oil

   Any of your favorite essential oils, if desired

Instructions

1. Combine almond oil, beeswax, coconut oil, and shea butter together.

2. Melt in a double boiler over low heat. Stir from time to time.

3. Take off from heat and set aside, once melted.

4. Add your favorite essential oil(s) and vitamin E oil.

5. Stir to incorporate.

6 Transfer into a glass jar, set aside until mixture solidifies.

7. Cover and store in a cool, dry place.

8. Apply twice daily, morning and night after face wash.

NOTE: Cream will stay for as long as 3 months.

Homemade Hi-C Anti Aging Facial Serum

This rich in natural vitamin C facial serum destroys wrinkles and reverses damage to the skin. It is also used to strengthen the barrier response of the skin, build collagen, reduce inflammation and many more.

Ingredients

1/4 cup aloe vera gel

2 teaspoons natural vitamin c powder

1 tablespoon fresh hibiscus petals or 1/2 tablespoon dried Hibiscus flowers

1/4 teaspoons vitamin E, if desired

Instructions

1. Mix dried hibiscus with aloe gel together.

2. Transfer aloe gel mixture into an electric blender or food processor.

3. Blend until the hibiscus changes to a pink-like color, for 5 to 10 times.

4. Set aside to extract favorable flavors, for 30 minutes.

5. Use a cloth/mesh strainer, strain aloe gel by squeezing it out from the hibiscus.

NOTE: You can straight twice, just to make sure you strained well.

6. Mix in vitamin C into the mixture slowly into the aloe vera gel mixture.

7. Stir well until natural vitamin C powder is well incorporated into the mixture.

8. Transfer into a dark bottle and lock lid in place.

NOTE: The dark bottle helps to keep the sun out, and preserve the longevity of vitamin C in the recipe.

9. Refrigerate bottle.

10. After toning and cleansing your face apply the serum to your décolleté, neck and face. Then moisturize your face.

NOTE: The vitamin E is a good combination with Vitamin C, and it also prevents the vitamin C in the recipe, from oxidizing so fast.

Mocha Mud Mask Anti Aging Recipe

Preparation Time: 2 minutes

Cook Time: 15 minutes

This mud mask energizes

Ingredients

1 tbsp cocoa powder

1 tsp coffee, finely ground

1 tbsp Bentonite clay

Few tsps of water

Instructions

1. In a plastic bowl, Toss in the cocoa powder, ground coffee and betonite clay.

2. Toss in sufficient water for a fine paste.

3. Using a wooden spoon stir mixture together until a paste-like consistency has been reached.

NOTE: Make sure you make use of a wooden spoon and a plastic bowl. Metals are not allowed with this recipe.

4. Apply using clean hands to rub on your chest and the face.

5. Allow mud mask to stay and dry for 15 minutes after application to the skin area.

6. Wash mask off, and then massage coffee into your skin, gently to exfoliate.

Anti Aging Serum Recipe

Ingredient

  2 tablespoons rosehip seed oil

  10 drops of cypress essential oil

  2 tablespoons sweet almond oil

  7 drops of frankincense essential oil

  10 drops of geranium essential oil

  2 oz. glass bottle.

Instructions

1. Combine rosehip seed oil, cypress essential oil, sweet almond oil, frankincense essential oil, and geranium essential oil.

2. Stir till a fine consistency is reached.

3. Transfer into a glass bottle.

4. Shake vigorously before use twice daily.

NOTE: Just a little amount just to cover your face and neck.

CHAPTER SIX - ORGANIC SKIN AND BEAUTY RECIPES TO FIGHT ACNE, BLEMISHES AND SPOTS

Your skin is in love with you and you are in love with your skin. Your skin is a loyal friend and you are a proud friend to your skin also. This beautiful relationship goes on for a while...

One day you wake up to discover that acne appears and damages the cordial relationship you have built with your skin over time.

Suddenly you start to hate and resent your skin. What is the next line of action? How can this love and friendship be restored?

It is not farfetched! The answer is not in harsh store bought chemicals. Simple answer... GO ORGANIC!

You will get maximum results if you start treating and handling your skin the right way.

DIY Acne Mask Recipe

Ingredients

2 tbsps apple cider vinegar

2 tbsps bentonite clay

Instructions

1. Combine ingredients well until thoroughly mixed.

NOTE: When well mixed, the mask will become thick

2. Avoid your eye area when applying to the face.

3. Leave on the face to dry for 10 to 20 minutes.

NOTE: If you have a skin that is sensitive, leave it for approximately 10 minutes.

Apple cider vinegar Acne Recipe

A bacteria killer, it eliminates acne causing bacteria and the pH of your skin gets balanced also. An astringent known to dry out too much oil on the skin.

Ingredients

3 tbsps fresh water

1 tbsp apple cider vinegar (pure & unfiltered)

Instructions

1. In a small bowl, combine water and apple cider vinegar together.

2. Mix well.

3. Wash your face well.

4. Place a cotton ball into the mixture gently, and apply vinegar soaked cotton ball on affected skin area, blemishes and acne.

5. Leave on your face 10 minutes before washing off thoroughly.

NOTE: You can leave it over the night and can be reapplied anytime in the day; this can be done many times.

6. After you wash off, moisturize your face.

Honey and Yogurt/Milk Spot Remover Mask

Ingredients

1 tbsp honey (raw & natural)

1 tbsp yogurt or milk (plain low-fat or full-fat)

Instructions

1. Set refrigerated milk or yogurt aside to cool properly.

2. Combine yogurt/milk with honey in a small bowl.

3. Mix thoroughly until well combined.

4. Wash your face and pat dry.

5. Apply by patting a thick layer of the mask on your face.

NOTE: For desired thickness, allow first layer dry before adding another layer. Repeat process until desired thickness is reached.

6. Leave on for 10 to 15 minutes to dry.

7. Wash your face, dry gently with a wash cloth to get rid of dead skin that has been loosened.

8. Apply moisturizer.

NOTE: You can use any plain full fat or low fat yogurt or milk, but do not use anything skimmed.

Honey with Cinnamon Face Mask

Ingredients

1 tsp cinnamon

2 tbsps honey

Instructions

1. Combine cinnamon and honey together in a bowl.

2. Mix together until well combined.

NOTE: A paste-like consistency should be reached.

3. Wash your face well, pat dry and apply mask to your face or area affected with spots.

4. Leave on for 10 to 15 minutes.

5. Wash face thoroughly and dry your face.

Papaya Acne Fighting Recipe

Ingredient

1 papaya, fresh

Instructions

1. Using a mortar and pestle or an electric blender, blend or grind the papaya flesh well adding a very small amount of water to form a paste.

NOTE: Add little water at a time, so as not to flood your mixture.

2. Keep blending until a paste-like consistency is reached.

3. Wash your face and pat dry.

4. Apply a thick layer to the affected areas or your face.

5. Leave on your face for 15 to 20 minutes.

6. Wash off from face and dry your face.

7. Apply moisturizer.

Egg whites Scar fading Mask

A simple and purse friendly way to remove scars and fight acne.

Ingredients

Washcloth

2 -3 egg whites (yolks removed)

Bowl

Instructions

1. Boil eggs until well cooked.

2. Set aside to cool, and then peel.

3. Remove yolks from egg whites.

4. Whisk egg whites until a frothy consistency is reached.

5. Set aside for 2-3 minutes.

6. Wash your face and pat dry.

7. Apply a thick layer of the mask to the affected area/spot/scar with the tips of your fingers.

NOTE: a) Clean your hands before application. b) Apply in succession, first layer dries out first before adding another layer. 3-4 layers should be okay for thick layer.

8. Leave on for 20 minutes to dry.

9. Wash face off, using warm water, and pat dry.

10 Moisturize your face accordingly.

Tea Tree Oil Remedy

This remedy works a natural magic that cuts through oily skin and skin cells that are dead and opens up the pores. Kills acne causing bacteria and prevents a reoccurrence.

Ingredients

1 tbsp tea tree oil

Cotton balls

9 tbsps Water, clean and fresh

Instructions

1. Combine water and tea tree oil together in a bowl.

2. Mix together until well combined.

3. Wash your face well, pat dry and apply remedy to your face or area affected with spots slowly, using cotton balls.

4. Apply moisturizer after application.

NOTE: a) You can make your mix stronger by changing the ratio of tea tree oil to water slightly. But don't start in a rush. Change preparation ratio slightly only after having used this mixture's ratio consistently for a minimum of a week. b) Aloe vera gel can be used as a substitute for water.

Orange Peel Paste Mask

Ingredients

2 Orange peels

Water, fresh and clean

Instructions

1. Using a mortar and pestle or an electric blender, blend or grind the orange peels adding a small amount of water to form a paste.

NOTE: Add little water at a time, so as not to flood your mixture.

2. Keep blending until a paste-like consistency is reached.

3. Wash your face and pat dry.

4. Apply a thick layer to the affected areas or your face.

5. Leave on your face for 20 to 25 minutes.

6. Wash off from face and dry your face.

7. Apply moisturizer.

Banana Peel Miracle

Ingredients

1 banana peel

Instructions

1. Separate peels from banana.

2. Apply by rubbing peels in circular motions over your face.

3. Leave on face for 30 minutes.

4. Wash off.

Honey & Strawberries Mix

Ingredients

2 tsps of raw honey

3 clean & fresh strawberries

Clean water

Instructions

1. Wash Strawberries and make sure they are clean.

2. Grind/pound strawberries well, adding very few drops of water.

NOTE: Don't over pound

3. Combine honey and mashed strawberries together.

4. Mix thoroughly until well combined.

5. Wash your face and pat dry.

6. Apply a thick layer to the affected areas or your face.

7. Leave on your face for 20 minutes.

6. Wash off from face with warm water and dry your face.

NOTE: Use 2 times weekly for 1 month or more.

Baking Soda Facial Mask

Baking soda also known as Sodium bicarbonate is known to exfoliate the skin, fight off bacteria and fungus, and also help to dry off excess skin oil. Your skin becomes glamorous and tender.

Ingredients

Fresh water

1 box baking soda

Instructions

1. Combine same amounts of water and baking soda together.

2. Stir to combine until a paste-like consistency is reached.

3. Wash face and pat dry.

4. Apply by massaging baking soda mask on your face and affected areas for 2 minutes. Move in circles as you apply.

5. Allow to dry for 15 to 20 minutes before washing off and pat drying gently.

NOTE: Use warm water to wash off.

6. Apply moisturizer.

Aloe Gel Acne Remedy

Ingredients

Aloe vera gel

Instructions

1. Wash and pat dry your face.

2. Apply a thick layer of aloe gel to the spot and other affected areas or your face.

3. Leave on your face for 10 minutes.

4. Wash off from face with warm water and dry your face.

Lemon Juice Touch

Ingredients

1 tbsp lemon juice, just squeezed

Yogurt, if desired

Cotton balls, if desired

Instructions

1. Combine yogurt and lemon juice together.

2. Stir to combine until well mixed.

3. Wash face and pat dry.

4. Apply by dipping cotton balls into yogurt/lemon mixture and rub on acne and other affected skin areas.

5. Wash off and pat dry gently.

NOTE: Use warm water to wash off.

Baking Soda Facial Scrub

Ingredients

1/8 cup fresh water

1/2 cup baking soda

Instructions

1. Combine water and baking soda together.

2. Stir to combine until a paste-like consistency is reached.

3. Wash face and pat dry.

4. Apply by massaging in the baking soda mask into your face and affected areas for 5 to 6 minutes.

NOTE: Move in circles as you apply.

5. Wash off and pat dry gently.

NOTE: Use warm water to wash off.

6. Apply moisturizer.

Garlic Natural Remedy

Ingredients

Aloe vera gel

2-3 cloves of garlic

Instructions

1. Pound the cloves of garlic until well mashed.

2. Measure in the aloe vera gel. Set aside to soak for 10 minutes.

3. Mash well until well mixed.

4. Dip cotton pad into the garlic juice and apply to spots/blemishes and acnes.

TIP: You can use remedy daily.

Steam Face Treatment

Steam helps to open up the skin and remove dirt, impurity that is beneath the skin. Steam alone works fine, but you can use this treatment before applying some other organic beauty treatments. The steam helps to clear the way for the other beauty treatments or recipes to do this its work effectively.

Ingredients

1 pot water

1 towel

1 large bowl

Instructions

1. Bring a pot of water to boiling.

2. Transfer water into the bowl.

3. Set aside for few minutes to lose a little bit of heat.

4. Set your face above the bowl, stopping short a little distance from the bowl.

5. To trap the steam and get maximum results; with the towel, cover your head, neck region and the bowl together.

NOTE: Drape towel in such a way that you contain as much of the steam as possible within the towel confinement.

6. Continue treatment for 10 to 15 minutes before pat drying your face.

TIP: You can do this every night or every morning or as needed.

Sugar Acne Fighting Scrub

Ingredients

Makes: 4 half pint jars

   1 ½ cups white sugar

   2-3 tbsps coarse sea salt

   1 ½ cups (light or dark) brown sugar

   10 tbsps pure vanilla extract

   1/2 cup (approx.) olive oil

   1 whole vanilla bean, if desired, (with caviar scrapped out)

Instructions

1. Combine white sugar, coarse sea salt, brown sugar and vanilla bean together.

2. Mix mixture thoroughly

3. In a liquid measuring cup, measure out two cups of this sugar/salt mixture.

NOTE: Press the mixture down to fill all air spaces in the measuring cup.

4. Toss olive oil over the measuring cup mixture and let it be absorbed by half the mixture.

5. Leave small layer on the top and spoon in 4 or 5 tbsps of vanilla extract into the mixture and stir to combine.

6. Transfer into smaller jars for use.

Oatmeal Booster

Ingredients

1 serving of oatmeal

2 tbsps honey, raw

Water

Instructions

1. Follow preparation instructions on the box of oatmeal; prepare oatmeal.

2. Take off from heat.

3. Measure in the honey.

4. Stir to incorporate honey into oatmeal well.

5. Set aside to cool to room temperature.

NOTE: Be sure it has really cooled.

6. Apply on skin and leave for 20 to 30 minutes to dry.

7 Wash off with warm water and pat dry.

Mint Fresh Relief

Ingredients

1 heaping handful of mint leaves, fresh

Instructions

1. In an electric blender, blend fresh mint leaves.

2. Blend until well mashed up.

3. Wash face and pat dry.

4. Apply crushed mint juice and leaves on your face.

5. Leave on for 5 to 10 minutes before washing with cold water.

6. Pat dry.

Honey & Avocado Face mask

Ingredients

1 tbsp of honey

1 avocado

Instructions

1. Remove the inside part of the avocado and pound it.

2. Stir mashed avocado inside with honey.

3. Keep pounding and stirring until a paste-like consistency is reached.

4. Wash your face and pat dry.

5. Apply honey and avocado face mask to your face.

6. Leave on 15 to 20 minutes.

7. Wash off with warm water and pat dry gently.

8. Moisturize your skin.

Potato Face Mask

Ingredients

1 potato, raw

Instructions

1. In a grater, grate potato.

2. Grate until well mashed up.

3. Wash face and pat face until almost dry.

4. Apply juice and pulp onto your face; moving in circles as you apply.

5. Leave on for 15 to 30 minutes to dry.

6. Wash off with warm water.

7. Pat dry.

Acne Spot Treatment

Ingredients

Brewer's yeast

Few tsps of water

1 squeeze of lemon juice

Instructions

1. Combine yeast, water and lemon juice together.

2. Mix to combine until paste-like consistency is reached.

3. Wash face and pat dry.

4. Apply the paste directly on your spots or blemishes.

5. Leave on for 8 to 10 minutes and covering with a bandage.

Tea Time

Recipe decreases skin oil, skin bacteria and inflammation. For topical use and can also be ingested to detoxify the body.

Ingredients

1 green tea bag or 2 tsps loose organic tea leaves

1/2 cup fresh water

Instructions

1. Bring water to a boil in a pot over medium heat.

2. Place tea leaves or tea bags in a bowl and pour the hot water on it.

3. Set aside for 4 to 5 minutes to release tea flavors.

4. Using mesh strainer or cheesecloth, strain out the leaves and set aside tea liquid to cool.

5. Transfer into a glass spray bottle and apply to your face lightly.

TIP: You can rinse off if you want to, and you can also leave on.

CHAPTER SEVEN - SEA SALT TREATMENTS FOR ORGANIC SKIN AND HAIR BEAUTY ROUTINES

Balancing Mask

Corrects irritation and breakouts, soothes and calms the skin. Helps to balance skin oil production also.

Ingredients

2 tsps finely ground sea salt

4 tsps honey, raw

Instructions

1. Combine honey and salt together in a small bowl.

2. Stir well to combine until a paste like consistency is reached.

3. Wash and pat dry skin.

4. Apply to the skin.

NOTE: Do not make mistakes of applying on the eyes.

5. Leave on for 10-15 minutes before washing with warm water.

TIP: a) Before washing your face, use a warm washcloth on your face; to massage your face for 30 seconds. b) Move your hands in circular movements.

Tender Body Scrub

Ingredients

1/4 cup salt

10 drops of your favorite essential oil

1/2 cup softened coconut oil or olive oil

Instructions

1. Combine salt and oil together

2. Stir well until a thick paste-like consistency is reached.

3. Measure in the essential of your choosing and stir to incorporate.

4. Wash face and pat dry.

5. Apply using a wash cloth or your palms to tenderly scrub your skin moving in circles.

Oil Removing Facial Toner

This facial toner helps to clean pores and drastically reduce oil production and fight bacteria.

Ingredients

1 tsp sea salt

4 oz. clean water.

Instructions

1. Bring water to boiling and set aside until warm.

2. Combine warm water and salt together.

3. Mix until the salt dissolves.

4. Transfer into a spray bottle.

5. Spritz on your face.

Relaxing Salt Bath

Ingredients

1/3 cup salt

1 full tub of warm water.

Instructions

1. Swish sea salt into the bath tub filled with warm water to dissolve.

2. Soak for 15-30 minutes.

Aloe Gel Lavender Scrub

Ingredients

1/2 cup salt

1/4 cup olive oil

1/4 cup aloe vera gel

1 tbsps of lavender flowers, dried.

Instructions

1. Combine salt, oil and aloe vera gel together.

2. Mix until a thick paste-like consistency is reached.

NOTE: if mixture is too dry, add little oil more.

3. Wash face and pat dry.

4. Apply using a wash cloth or your palms to tenderly scrub your skin moving in circles.

Teeth Whitening Treatment

Ingredients

2 tsps baking powder

1 tsp salt

Instructions

1. Combine baking powder and salt together.

2. Mix until properly combined.

3. Wet toothbrush with water and dip into baking powder mixture.

4. Apply brushing your teeth as you would with regular toothpaste.

TIP: You can add a little bit of your regular toothpaste with this mixture.

Dandruff Fighting Scalp Treatment

This recipe combats fungi and absorbs excessive moisture on the skin.

Ingredients

1-2 tsps salt.

Few drops of water

Instructions

1. Apply by sprinkling salt on your scalp.

2. Moisten your hands with water and massage scalp thoroughly with wet hands for 10-15 minutes.

3. Wash, pat dry your hair. Apply hair conditioning cream.

Nail Brightening Miracle

Ingredients

1 tsp salt

1 tsp baking soda

1 tsp lemon juice

1/2 cup water.

Instructions

1. Warm water in a small pot.

2. In a small bowl, combine salt, lemon juice, warm water and baking soda together.

3. Dip your nails into the warm water salt solution for 10 minutes.

4. After 10 minutes, your nails should be scrubbed using soft brush.

5. Rinse your hands and apply moisturizer.

All-Natural Mouth Wash

Ingredients

1/2 tsp salt

1/2 tsp baking soda

1/4 cup water

Instructions

1. Combine baking soda, salt and water together.

2. Mix well until the salt is dissolved in the mixture.

3. Pour a little of the solution into your mouth, swish around and gargle.

4. Spit out and then wash your mouth.

CHAPTER EIGHT - ORGANIC SKIN AND BEAUTY RECIPES FOR CLEARING THE SKIN

Lemon Skin Clearing Treat

Ingredients

Freshly squeezed lemon juice

1-2 tbsps honey, raw

Instructions

1. Extract juice from lemon.

2. Combine honey and lemon juice. Stir until consistent.

3. Wash face and pat dry.

4. Apply to the neck region and the face.

5. Leave on for 15-20 minutes.

6. Wash off with warm water and pat face dry.

7. Rub slices of cucumber on your skin to moisturize and soften your skin.

TIP: You can give your skin this treat daily or thrice weekly.

Honey Skin Clearing Treat

Ingredients

2 tsps milk

1 tsp honey

1 tsp gram flour

Instructions

1. Combine milk, honey and flower together.

2. Stir together until a paste like consistency is reached.

3. Wash and pat dry face.

4. Rub on your face and leave to dry for 20 minutes.

5. Wash your face with warm water and pat dry.

TIP: Apply once weekly for a clear and bright skin.

Turmeric Skin Clearing Treat

Ingredients

1 tbsp turmeric powder

few tsps pinepple juice

Instructions

1. Combine turmeric and pineapple together and mix well.

2. Wash face and pat dry.

3. Apply the paste to the neck and face and leave for 15 to 20 minutes.

4. Wash with warm water and pat dry.

TIP: Use 2-3 times weekly.

Baking Soda Skin Clearing Treat

Ingredients

1 tsp baking soda

1 tsp water

1 tsp lemon juice.

Instructions

1. Combine ingredients together.

2. Mix until paste-like consistency is reached.

3. Wash your face and pat dry.

4. Apply as a mask for exfoliating the skin.

5. Leave to dry and wash off with warm water, pat dry.

TIP: Use 2-3 times weekly.

Aloe Vera Skin Clearing Treat

This recipe helps new skin cells to grow and moisturizes the skin

Ingredients

Aloe vera gel

Cotton ball

Instructions

1. Wash and pat dry your face.

2. Use cotton ball to apply aloe gel on your face.

3. Leave on for 30 minutes.

4. Wash off with warm water.

TIP: Once every day for 5 months.

Papaya Skin Clearing Treat

Ingredients

Ripe papaya, chopped

1 tsp sandalwood powder

1 tsp honey

Instructions

1. Combine ingredients together.

2. Blend mixture until a paste like consistency is reached.

3. Wash and pat dry your face.

4. Apply to the face and leave on for 30-60 minutes.

5. Wash off and dry.

6. Follow with rose water to the face.

TIP: This should be used once weekly for a tremendous quantifiable change in skin tone.

Cucumber Skin Clearing Treat

Ingredients

1 tbsp of cucumber juice

1 tbsp of lemon juice

Instructions

1. Combine ingredients together.

2. Stir until well combined.

3. Wash and pat dry your skin.

4. Apply mixture to affected skin area, leave to dry; and then wash off.

TIP: Use daily.

Walnut Skin Clearing Treat

Ingredients

2 tsps walnut powder

2 tbsps plain yogurt

Instructions

1. Come both ingredients together.

2. Stir well until paste-like consistency is reached.

3. Wash and pat dry your face.

4. Apply to the face and leave on till paste dries off, for 60 minutes.

5. Wash off with warm water and dry your face by patting.

TIP: a) This should be used once weekly for a tremendous quantifiable change in skin tone.

b) Eat 2-3 walnuts with 1 glass of milk each morning. Mix two teaspoons of walnut powder with two tablespoons of plain yogurt to make a paste. Apply this paste on.

END

Thank you for reading my book. I hope you enjoyed it? Thanks!

Jacqueline S Mendez